Detox:
ACHIEVE A FLAT BELLY THE NATURAL WAY

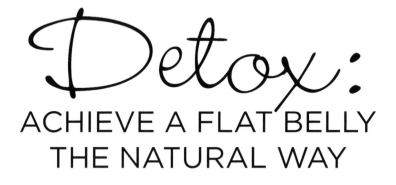

KIKS SEAH

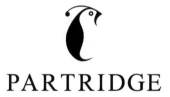

PARTRIDGE

To order additional copies of this book, contact
Toll Free +65 3165 7531 (Singapore)
Toll Free +60 3 3099 4412 (Malaysia)
orders.singapore@partridgepublishing.com

www.partridgepublishing.com/singapore

LEGAL & DISCLAIMER

The information contained in this book is not designed to replace or take the place of any form of medicine or professional medical advice. The information in this book has been provided for educational and entertainment purposes only.

The information contained in this book has been compiled from sources deemed reliable, and it is accurate to the best of the Author's knowledge; however, the Author cannot guarantee its accuracy and validity and cannot be held liable for any errors or omissions. Changes are periodically made to this book. You must consult your doctor or get professional medical advice before using any of the suggested remedies, techniques, or information in this book.

Upon using the information contained in this book, you agree to hold harmless the Author from and against any damages, costs, and expenses, including any legal fees potentially resulting from the application of any of the information provided by this guide. This disclaimer applies to any damages or injury caused by the use and application, whether directly or indirectly, of any advice or information presented, whether for breach of contract, tort, negligence, personal injury, criminal intent, or under any other cause of action.

You agree to accept all risks of using the information presented inside this book. You need to consult a professional medical practitioner in order to ensure you are both able and healthy enough to participate in this program.

CONTENTS

INTRODUCTION

Is there a miracle solution to help someone's belly melt away? Don't we all wish that such a solution exists? The truth is that you have to be actively involved in this process and be ready to make the sacrifices required. There is no short cut to it if we want to do the **natural** way.

This book will explain why abdominal area often seems to be the target area for weight gain. We offer you several different natural methods to decrease your belly fat, and intentionally avoid those options that are not natural. By working on decreasing your belly fat the correct and natural way, you will have more chances to take care of the problem for good.

By utilizing some simple eating tips, you will realize how quickly you can transform your belly and your life! As with so many things, consistency is the key.

We will dedicate a chapter about health benefits and you will see the importance of losing this fat around your belly. You can share these benefits with your partner, your loved ones, and your friends if you still find yourself in need of additional motivation. However, as with any diet, exercise plan, or any major change in your life or way of living, you should always consult your primary care physician (if you have one). Your primary care physician knows your medical history better than anyone else.

The benefits of having a smaller and trimmer belly are extensive, and you will soon be convinced that it is imperative that you put in all the necessary effort to get where you want and need to be, when it comes to the size of your stomach.

You will learn many exercises you can perform at home or in the gym to assist in losing that unwanted extra fat in your belly area, as well as strengthening your abdominal muscles. We are all familiar with the famous sit-ups, but are you doing them right? And you will learn other activities that you can do that are very efficient in helping you to lose fat in that very specific area. You can reach your goals by keeping yourself focused and combining a regular exercise plan with a healthy diet. Make these exercises as fun as possible; listening to your favorite music or doing them with a friend or workout partner. You will be surprised to know how many possibilities there are to help you slim away that belly of yours. Start today and notice the results very soon!

Finally, in order to keep your belly fat down and still enjoy a good meal, you should equip yourself with a variety of healthy recipes. In order to cook healthier, choose the ingredients carefully. It does not mean that the food you eat should taste bland. You will be able to keep yourself motivated and focused if you find delicious and easy recipes to cook. It can also be fun to cook with your children or your spouse, so make sure you involve everyone that can help you achieve your goals, or even better, make it a family journey towards health.

Soon enough, it will become second nature for you to pick the right ingredients to help your stomach stay flat. Also, you will learn how to replace healthier ingredients in your recipe books. Be creative, and enjoy your meals at the table, combine other tips given earlier in the book to keep the weight off. Bon appetit!

Chapter 1

WHERE DOES THE BELLY FAT COME FROM?

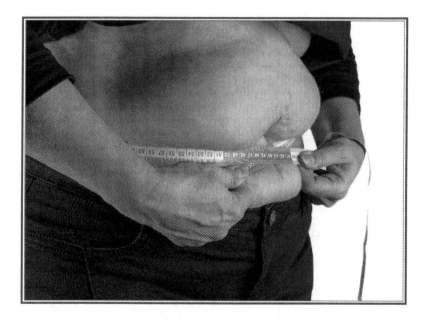

For some of us when we gain weight, it lodges right down around our belly area. It can be quite frustrating at times, as it seems to be an eternal struggle. Let's first try to understand why the fat accumulation is always in the stomach area instead of other areas.

Hormones are driving most of the changes in our bodies and our fat storage. Fat bellies can be seen on thin individuals as well as heavier individuals.

PHYSIOLOGICAL CAUSES

First, belly fat has a lot to do with hormones.

When you ingest food, your body starts breaking fats down and transforming it into energy. Glucose is the main source of energy for your body, and insulin is the hormone secreted to the pancreas responsible for carrying the glucose through your bloodstream. Sometimes the insulin transports the energy, or glucose, and it is used right away, and sometimes it is stored in the body. So if you eat a meal rich in carbs or glucose (sugar), your insulin level goes up. This means that if you don't expend that energy right away, the excess will be stored away for later use in the form of fat.

Additionally, depending on what food you are choosing, your hormone insulin can react slightly differently. If your diet is rich in refined carbs such as white bread, white rice and other simple sugars, the level of insulin will go up. As a consequence, when the insulin level goes up, so does the belly fat. So, you should favor foods higher in proteins, healthy fats, and fiber to help the insulin and blood sugar levels go down.

The stress hormones are another type of hormones that can significantly determine the percentage of belly fat in your body, as they play a role in determining the amount of belly fat your body can produce and store. If you are stressed out, your poor body will produce adrenaline, a hormone that can actually release stored energy as needed. During the release of this stored energy, fatty acids will also be released, as well as the hormone cortisol, which helps the fatty acids recuperate. The problem arises when the hormone cortisol does not transport the fatty acids back, but instead concentrate its activity in your abdomen area. Simply put, being overstressed equals storing additional fat in your belly area. However, it is important to understand that cortisol is an important hormone to help your body function normally. It is important to control the production of cortisol, and to keep it at an acceptable level by making sure you get enough sleep and trying to control the physical and/or emotional stresses to which you are exposing your body.

Again, this is a simplified explanation and your belly area is not the only part of your body where your hormones can influence the storage of fat, but it is an area that is more subject to and more sensitive to it.

HEREDITY AND MEDICAL CONDITIONS

Our genes can also have an important influence and impact on the size of our belly. Yes, you might have a predisposition for a larger belly due to your genetic history. And for a lot of people, especially men, large bellies can be related to lifestyle.

Certain medical conditions can also make you more prone to developing a bigger stomach area. Thyroid dysfunction is one of these —the hormones secreted by the thyroid gland regulate some of the activities in your body, and if this gland does not work properly, it can lead to weight gain or other health problems. In fact, when the thyroid does not sufficiently create the needed hormones, the individual will most likely gain weight.

Cushing's syndrome is another condition that can be responsible for fat bellies. This is due to the adrenal glands producing too much cortisol.

Depression can also be a major factor in weight gain, as some individuals can be prone to "eating their emotions".

If you are experiencing any issues with your thyroid, or any other health issues in general, make sure you consult with your primary care physician. They will be able to give you the best advice regarding your health, as they will know your medical history better than anyone.

GENDER DIFFERENCES

Men and women store or gain weight in different areas. First, it is a fact that women carry a larger amount of fat than men. They are also more prone to storing the extra fat in their hips, legs, and buttocks areas. Men, on the other hand, have a tendency to store that unwanted fat in the upper part of their body. The insulin production as explained above performs differently in and men's and women's bodies. So, this can explain why you see the belly fat more frequently in men.

Also, both genders burn fat differently. When dieting, women will lose weight in the upper part of their body first unless they are pregnant or breastfeeding. In general, females will be able to burn calories and fat easier when they do physical activities.

Just because men in general might have more of a problem with fat bellies than women, it does not mean that women never experience this problem. During menopause, for example, many women will experience body changes, and while even avoiding weight gain can still experience changes in their body proportions.

So, we can see that the hormonal disposition of our bodies can influence how we gain weight and where. Men produce testosterone, and if this particular hormone gets low, it is associated with larger bellies. For woman, estrogen will contribute to smaller waists, as it does counter-act the storage of calories and fat in the belly area. Finally, adrenaline and noradrenaline are hormones released during intensified physical activity and will behave differently depending on your gender. Either way, these hormones will help to burn visceral belly fat (deep stomach fat).

Chapter 2

FLAT STOMACH NATURAL SOLUTIONS

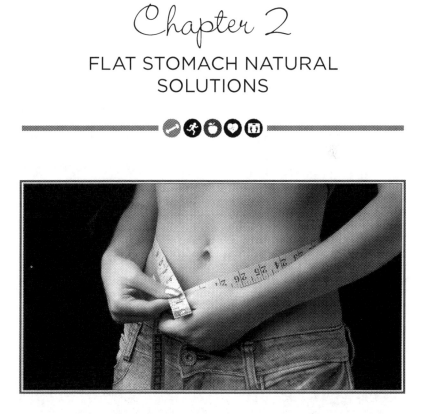

To create calorie deficiency, the body must burn more calories than it takes in. Average / moderate active females require 2000 calories/ day. Average/ moderate active males require 2600 calories/ day. Eating below 1200 calories/day is extremely unhealthy.

Our eating habits are certainly one of the most influential factors in determining whether or not we will be successful in losing the unwanted weight in our belly region. Those people who eat healthy breakfast tend to weigh less than those who do not. Switching sodas for water or other 'no calorie' beverage reduces overall calorie intake. We should pick food that are high in fiber, protein, and essential minerals. Diet rich in fiber and protein could lose fat without exercises. Protein is helpful in fighting insulin resistance.

Listed below are some foods to favor or foods to avoid in your pursuit of a slimmer belly.

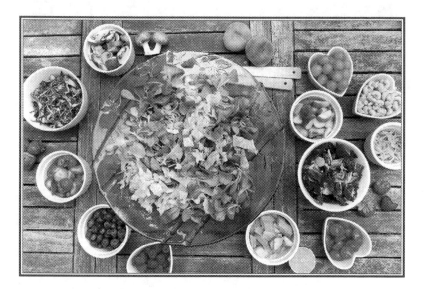

FOODS TO FAVOR

- Proteins (Whole eggs, seafood --fish such as salmon and tuna with monounsaturated fats, lean meats, poultry)

- Soy products

- Low fat dairy products (cheese, yoghurt, milk)

- Whole grains (cereals, oatmeal)

- Vegetables (especially dark green, avocados, tomatoes, celery best eaten raw etc.)

- Coconut oil **

- Olive oil

- Nuts i.e. almonds, pecans, walnuts, seeds (avoid the salty ones which can cause your blood pressure to increase)

- Fruits (water melons, apples, bananas)

- Beans and legumes eg. Pinto beans and green beans (high in fiber & protein)

It was researched that fiber –rich apples or pinto beans reduce visceral fat by a few percent / year.

- Peanut butter is a good source of protein and niacin (1 tbsp. a day max)

- Iced tea (preferably green tea).

- Hot water with lemon and honey in the morning

- Salad before lunch and dinner

- 1 tablespoon of vinegar everyday (Apparently a Japanese Studies showed obese people who consumed a couple of tablespoons of vinegar everyday for 8 weeks showed dramatic reduction in visceral body fat. It seems that the acetic acid in vinegar produces fat- burning protein).

Coconut oil *is known to act as an appetite suppressant. It also contains fatty acids that have been reported to help boost the metabolism, so the energy is distributed instead of stored in your body. Your cholesterol levels HDL (good cholesterol), will be increased when using coconut oil in your meal and the LDL (bad cholesterol) should decrease, which is another important and healthy advantage.*

FOODS TO AVOID

- Any sodas or sugary drinks (fruit juices, sport drinks, sugared coffee and teas)

- Refined sugars (cookies, cakes, table sugar, candies, syrup)

- Salty foods or "bag snacks" (chips, crackers etc.)

- Processed Foods (avoid as much as possible)

- High saturated fat food (such as fried food etc.)

- Starchy Vegetables (Corn, potatoes etc.)

- Deli meats

- Sauces (salad dressings and gravy etc.)

- Carbs (white breads, pastas, white rice)

- Beer

HERBS AND SPICES

If you are going to opt for natural ingredients to lose weight, you might seriously consider looking into the use of fresh herbs and spices to help you. Among the best and most efficient are ginger, ginseng, cinnamon, and cayenne pepper. This last spice works at boosting your metabolism, so you will burn calories and fat faster, and it can also act as an appetite suppressant. Try the cayenne pepper on your chicken and fish—it's delicious! Ginger is known to help your tissues burn more energy and more calories leading to weight loss and better control of your cholesterol. Cinnamon, is not only delicious in many meals and cereals, but it is also efficient on lowering your blood sugar level. Cinnamon is a good source of fiber and calcium as well. Ginseng is also great at boosting your immune system and increasing your endurance. Additionally, it has been reported that ginseng helps in controlling high blood pressure.

DIETING OPTIONS

You do not have to start following a specific or strict diet to necessarily lose the unwanted weight. You can start by combining several small changes, such as reducing the portions you eat at every meal. Eat less calories creating a Calorie Deficit. Cut down foods that are dense in calories such as butter, fruit juice and desserts. By cutting down certain foods and your daily caloric intake, you will be surprised at how much of an impact it can have on your belly and waist.

Don't go on an extreme diet. If you do, you might lose weight at first, but chances are you will soon feel frustrated and gain back to the original weight and possibly more. Be patient. Losing one or two pounds a week is perfect. Think about it in the long term, and in terms of your health, and not just a number on a scale.

There are numerous dieting options for you, and some will keep you away from the carbs completely, and others will encourage a high dose of proteins. There is no miracle solution. Simply choose the diet that seems to best fit your taste buds and needs. You can also talk to your primary care physician for additional advice.

Whether or not you are counting calories, it is a great idea to write down what you consume in a journal. A lot of people do not realize how the many little trivial "bites" they eat daily can add up, calorically speaking.

For example, if you are the cook in the family, I challenge you for one week to stop eating, tasting, or "grazing" upon whatever food you are cooking. This adds up! While it can be difficult to quantify (or keep track of) that extra piece of cheese you cut off for yourself while making your sandwich, or that extra piece of luncheon meat you eat when you are making your sandwich, trust that these aren't freebies…they add up! If you are cognitive of it and are making a serious effort to write down the food you put in your mouth every day, you will be surprised. Sometimes we end up eating even if we are not hungry. We eat by habit, we eat our emotions, or we eat simply because we are gathering with friends.

By keeping a journal, you will feel obligated to stop and think before you actually unwrap that candy bar or get up to get seconds. But the keys here are diligence, accuracy, and honesty. Remember, if you cheat, you are only cheating yourself.

CLEANSING OPTIONS

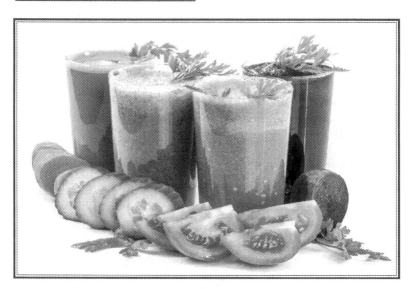

A cleansing diet is also an option, and there are several different kinds of cleansing diets. You will also find them listed under detox diets. Detoxifying your body is always a good idea once in a while to feel recharged and rejuvenated. It gives you sort of a fresh start, as you will deeply clean your insides - your pipes. It is almost like doing your spring cleaning in your house a few times a year. It is necessary... and then you can simply switch to maintenance. o, you can choose the juices or cleanser you prefer and adopt that method for a few days or as recommended. After that, you will need to make sure you keep consuming foods high in fiber and drink plenty of water, to help in keeping up regularly.

CREATING MEALS

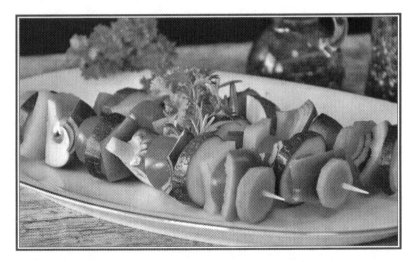

In order to lose weight and be satisfied, you need to eat a variety of foods so you do not get bored or frustrated. Be creative when you cook. Use healthy ingredients such as colorful vegetables, and add fresh herbs and spices for taste. Equip yourself with new recipe books and try to make your favorites using healthier ingredients. Buy a juicer so you can make fresh juices or a sherbet machines for healthy sweet treats. Remember that everything is about moderation and that you should not skip meals, but actually eat several small meals a day if possible. In fact, it is suggested that you eat 5 or 6 small meals a day might be the best solution, since it will help boost your metabolism which will then burn fat more efficiently.

Changing your eating habits

- Make sure you do sit at the table and enjoy your meal. You should not be rushed and you should try to eat as slowly as possible. When you chew your food longer, it aids digestion. By chewing your food properly, you will not feel bloated and your body will get the chance to absorb the nutrients better. This will also give you more of an opportunity to feel fuller quicker, and helps you to eat less.

- Eat small proportions of food every 2-3 hours if possible. This keeps the digestive system running smoothly.

- Avoid hanging around the fridge and eating because of boredom. Stay busy and hydrated. Remove junk food.

It is also important to make sure to keep healthy snacks handy readily available at all times. Whether it be at the office, between baseball practices, or after a workout, pack some fruits, nuts or yogurt. In this way you can avoid buying or choosing processed foods from the vending machine or convenience store, as well as never letting yourself get so hungry that you over- eat. These small snacks in between meals count as one of your five or six small meals you should eat daily. Take pleasure in knowing that you are helping to boost that metabolism!

STRESS MANAGEMENT

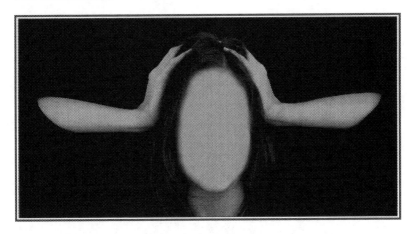

Stress will cause cortisol levels to rise, which will make fat loss more difficult. It can cause the body to hold on to fats.

Reduction in stress will improve sleep and will in turn reduce cortisol levels.

Here are some strategies below.

- Talk to friends.
- Find time to relax, and comforting activity to lessen stress levels like meditation.
- Take Vitamin C to counteract stress, and it is also useful for burning fat.

Chapter 3

BENEFITS OF A FLAT STOMACH

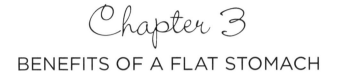

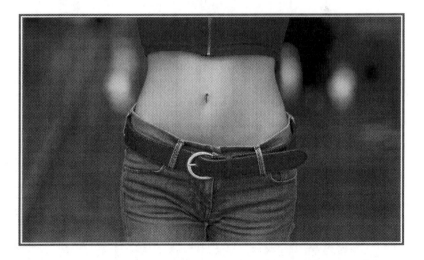

There are many benefits of losing weight. Some might be more related to your personal needs and desires, while others may be less obvious and be health related. Either way, working on a flat stomach is a great idea, as long as you are not under eating or trying to starve yourself, and also as long as you are making sure to get enough rest.

BOOSTING YOUR SELF-CONFIDENCE

No one likes having a big, flabby belly. Women want to wear that sexy dress they bought for New Year's and men want to be able to take off their shirts at the pool. It is easy to understand that when you look the way you want to look, and feel better about yourself, you have higher self-esteem. That self-esteem boost can manifest itself in many different ways—when you think about getting a promotion at work, compete in a beauty pageant or simply being back in the dating world.

By feeling better, and carrying less weight around, you will have more energy and be more efficient in your day to day life. You will feel more productive, and happier. Usually, when you lose weight, it's possible that you will breathe better, and even think more clearly and make better decisions.

BETTER POSTURE

Strengthening your core or abdominal area, can also help with your posture. Your stomach muscles will become stronger as you lose the weight and practice a regular program of exercise, and your flexibility can even be improved. When you don't work your abdominal muscles, your back does all of the work and you can develop back pain. By working on the muscles in your abdomen, you can decrease or eliminate any back pain you may be having.

IMPROVING MANY HEALTH CONDITIONS

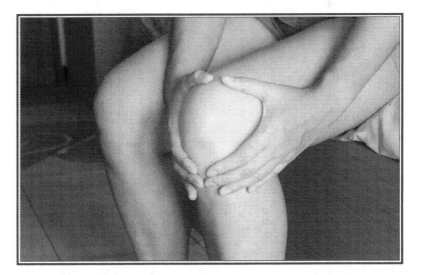

Unfortunately, we cannot choose which areas of our body lose weight the quickest. But losing weight, regardless in what part of your body, can have multiple health benefits. It is sometimes even recommended by your doctor to do so in order to avoid having to take medication, or simply to improve your general health. It is also important not to buy into the general way of thinking that a big belly comes with age. If you are motivated to improve your health and appearance, it is possible, and you should work on getting rid of that unwanted belly of yours.

Many diseases or medical conditions can be improved, prevented, or even eliminated by controlling your weight. Losing your belly fat can certainly help your digestive system to work better. It has also been proven that the fat deposit around your abdomen is directly linked to diabetes for certain individuals. If you are controlling your blood sugar level better, it could also reduce a condition named 'restless legs syndrome' associated with diabetes. Reducing your belly fat is also known to lessen your chances of heart disease, stroke, and heart attack. It can also help in controlling blood pressure and cholesterol (lower the good cholesterol – increasing the bad one).

Visceral fat is white fat expanding in the abdomen and wraps around the organs. And because it is so close to other organs in your body, it can greatly affect the mechanics of your body, or how your body works. Some types of cancer are more prevalent in individuals who have excess fat in the belly area, including: breast, pancreas, esophageal, and colon cancer. Be aware, also that a heavier weight can sometimes be a sign of a larger organ and should definitely be looked at by a health professional. Although your belly fat might be partially genetic, don't give up, and try to improve your health by losing the weight and keep your middle area trim.

A larger abdomen can also put extra pressure on your back and joints and can cause you a lot of discomfort, and those aches and pains can be greatly reduced by cutting down your belly fat. And logically, if you are not constantly experiencing pain when you are active, you will have a tendency to exercise more, it is a vicious-or healthy cycle. But initially, it may be necessary to take it slow and work through the aches in order to be able to get to the point where exercising is more of a pleasure and less of a…well…pain.

Simple changes in your hormones can also cause you to have a fatter belly area. For example, women can experience this when they reach menopause. Sometimes, the fat will accumulate in the abdominal area instead of the hips or thighs, but it depends on the individual. In both men and women however, it is more important than ever to keep yourself active as you get older, to decrease any chances of health problems as well as keeping yourself more agile and mobile.

Your sleep can also be greatly improved with regular exercise by losing the extra fat. If you are carrying excess weight, you are more prone to develop obstructive sleep apnea. This condition happens when the airway is blocked partially or completely during sleep. So, by sleeping better, it will help you feel more energized; and enables you to get up and start each day fresher, thus accomplish more, exercise more, and eventually maintain your desired weight.

Chapter 4

LOSE YOUR BELLY FAT BY EXERCISING

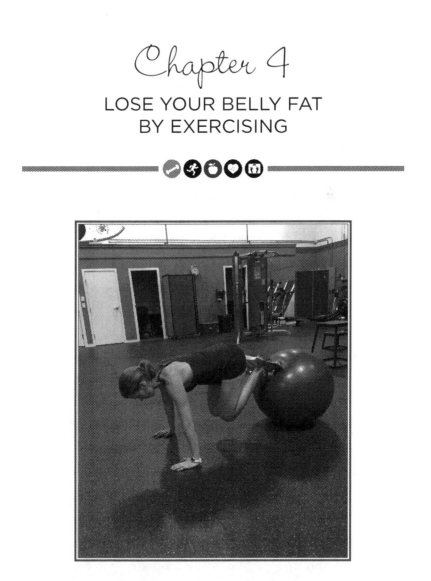

Losing fat without exercise will increase the risk of losing lean body mass, which will slow down the bodies' metabolism.

This will put the body into fat- storing mode. People who have lost body fat as well as muscle mass may notice that they do not have the muscle mass they had before. Then they over- eat, and repeat the cycle of filling up the body fat again.

By building muscle mass and bone strength, you help to increase your metabolism and burn more calories and fat. It is especially important to incorporate strength training into your life as you age because, unfortunately, as we age we will also lose muscle and lessen the amount of calories we burn daily. Again, it is all connected. And if you truly want to give yourself the best chance of losing that extra accumulation of fat around your belly, there is no easy fix. You have to incorporate strength training into your exercise routine. You also have to incorporate plenty of aerobic or cardiovascular activity.

So here you are, eating better, or at least changing a few of your eating habits and cutting out the foods you should be cutting out. You might lose a few pounds, and you should definitely start feeling at least a little better and healthier. But to be able to start seeing a difference in your abdominal area, you will also need to add a regular exercise routine to your new lifestyle.

It is important to understand here that cardiovascular exercise is vital to the elimination of belly fat. Sit-ups and other exercises that target the abdominal muscles are necessary to strengthen those muscles and eventually give you that six pack you are hoping for, if that is your goal. But if those muscles are covered in layer upon layer of fat, you are not going to be able to show off those strong abs you have worked so hard to develop.

Very simply put, when you get your heart pumping, and elevate your pulse, you will burn calories and eventually lose weight—provided you are burning more calories than you consume. There are many other factors and variables involved, but again, this is very simply put. That is the basic idea. Another factor in burning fat is your metabolism, and there are many methods of increasing your own metabolism like eating very small amounts up to six times a day, and getting enough sleep.

As far as strengthening your abdominal area, performing exercises that target these muscles will be the method by which you can tone and shape these muscles. With time and a continued fierce devotion to cardiovascular exercise, hopefully you will be able to see the results of your hard work and dedication.

Just like keeping a journal with your daily caloric intake, so should you with your exercising. If you make a conscious effort to write down your daily trips to the gym, whether it was a cardio day or a weight training day, muscles worked, and calories burned (you can invest in an inexpensive heart monitor), and your weight each day, you will be surprised at how motivating this can be. Also, in the same journal, document the days where you took the day off from exercising (because resting your body is important as well). There will be times when you will have that inner argument about whether or not you want to work out, and you do simply to be able to put it in the book, and you may even feel guilty if you don't! You can also keep track of which muscles you worked during your previous strength training session (you should allow 48 hours rest for your different muscles). The more you get involved in your own fitness, the more interested and motivated you will be. Journaling can also give you more specific information with which to work—you can look at what has been working for you, a certain week where you lost a few pounds, for example.

CARDIO ACTIVITIES

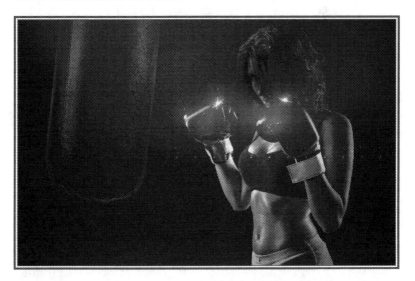

As stated earlier, cardio is fundamental to weight loss. It's very important to adopt an activity that will keep you interested and motivated in the long run, and one that you will maintain. You would want to make sure to choose an activity that you enjoy. Obviously not everyone enjoys the same things, but luckily the possibilities are extensive.

Some simple cardio exercises like jumping rope, sprinting and swimming help to burn extra calories. Running up and down the stairs 15 sets in a go is good cardio exercises. You should mix up the other types of exercises for your abdominals in order to avoid losing its effectiveness.

Some people enjoy the peace and solitude they find while running by themselves. Some people will feel more motivated if they exercise with a friend or a partner. In these cases, you can easily turn to activities like racquetball or tennis. Others may enjoy a larger group activity with great music like Zumba, or a body pump class, or even spinning. There are so many choices these days and you can inquire at the gym or recreational club to which you belong. Try them all if you like before making your choice. Pilates and yoga are also very popular, although they include a lot of stretching and can do you some good. You probably want to complement this activity with another more cardiovascular activity. Try kickboxing or martial arts. Also you could learn self-defence and gain some tight abs at the same time!

If you like the social aspect of playing sports, join a soft ball team, basketball team, or try some beach volleyball if you live in an accommodating climate. Any sport where you get your heart pumping will help you accomplish your goal. Also, if team sports is your cup of tea, you will hardly feel like you are working out and you will have a blast!

If on the other hand, if you are a loner when it comes to physical activity, no worries! There are plenty of activities from which to choose that can still help you get to your goal of losing that excess belly fat. Ride your bike or going for a jog is certainly a great way to burn calories. Swimming 10-20 laps every day at the community pool, will also help you achieve your goal. Why not take an extra-long walk 3 or 4 times a week with your favorite furry companion, or with your favorite tunes?

Finally, if you are a parent of young children and already have trouble keeping up with your busy schedule, think about creative ways to incorporate exercises into your life. You can of course, go out and play with your little ones. Help them practise for their next game or play Marco polo in the pool with them. Organize volleyball on the beach every weekend with friends and have adult and kids' tournament. Go outside with them also when it's time to build a snow man, a fort, or participate at a fun snow ball fight! Not only you will do yourself some good but you will also add family fun time in your agenda!

SIT-UPS

The wonderful thing about sit-ups is that you can do them anywhere. They can be very uncomfortable if done on a hard surface, but if you equip yourself with a yoga mat you do not have to wait until you are at the gym to do them, and you will not have any excuse not to do them on a regular basis. You can even do them while lying in bed and watching TV or in your living room, listening to your favorite music. Maybe you have a toddler crawling around that you constantly have to follow around and keep out of trouble? Get down on the floor with them and you will be amazed at the new interaction you can create while you exercise.

So, what is an efficient sit-up?

Your arms should either be folded across your chest, or behind your neck with your fingers laced behind your head where you can support your head. You should try as much as possible to use only your abdominal muscles to lift yourself up. As explained previously, sit-ups can potentially work on many muscles so they are a great addition to your workout routine.

The correct positon is to lay flat with your knees up and your feet flat on the ground. You will gently pull yourself up *slowly* until your eye contact is on your knees and you should aim for a ninety-degree angle. You should hold the position for a few seconds and then lower yourself *slowly* back into the starting position. Do as many as you can, increasing slightly each week. A variation of this exercise can be done by slightly twisting as you raise, and touching your elbow to the opposite knee, alternating sides, but keeping your feet flat on the ground. Like any other exercise, the important thing is to concentrate on your form and do them slowly.

CRUNCHES

Crunches sometimes get mixed up with sit-ups because the difference is very subtle. With crunches, you do not raise all the way up to the 90 degrees angle, nor do you go all the way back down to a flat position. The idea with crunches is to keep your abdominal muscles tensed the entire time.

EXAMPLE OF REVERSE CRUNCHES

Step 1: Lie down your body

Step 2: Raise legs to form 90 degrees angle between legs, and back lying on the ground.

Step 3: Place hands facing the ground on either side of your body.

Step 4: While raising your legs, inhale as much air as you can.

Step 5: Exhale and lower your legs back to starting position.

** Do not drop legs suddenly. Lower down your legs in a slow motion and exhale all the air intake. Do 15 to 20 repetition of exercises for better results.

EXAMPLE OF FULL PLANK EXERCISE

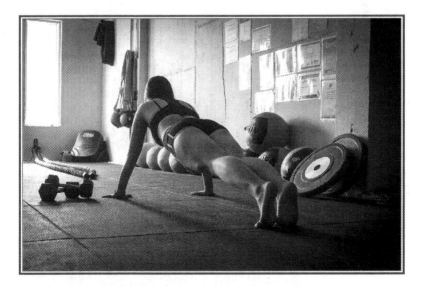

Step 1: Push Option position

Step 2: Bend elbows in 90 degrees

Step 3: Rest body weight on your forearms and hold your body weight.

Step 4: Align your body to form a straight line from shoulders to ankles. Hold your body in this position as long as you can.

Target: Hold body in this position for minimum of 1 minute.

SLEEP

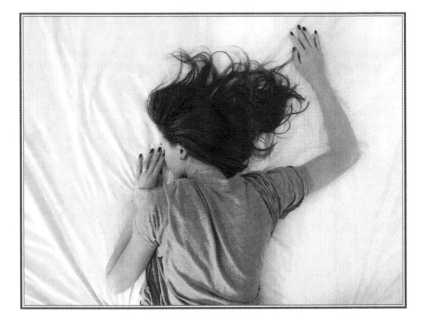

While sleeping is certainly not exercising, it is just as important to you in your quest to lose the fat around your belly area. On the more obvious level, sleep is essential for you to be able to function during the day and to have the energy to be able to work and exercise.

In a 2010 Wake Forest University Study, it concluded that people who sleep an average of 5 hours a night or less have a much harder time with the battle of the bulge. Lacking sleep induces hormone production and causes weight gain. Having less than 5 hours or more than 8 hours of sleep negatively impact fat loss.

It is recommended the optimum amount of sleep is 6-7 hours.

Managing sleep and eating timings regulate metabolism. On the not so obvious level, many studies show that you continue to burn fat as you sleep, and that the healing in your body and muscles occurs when you are asleep. So, you have to make sure to allow yourself to have enough sleep, and for some individuals this takes a very conscious effort.

$Chapter\ 5$

QUESTIONS AND ANSWERS

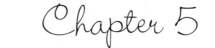

HOW CAN I TELL IF MY WAIST SIZE IS PROBLEMATIC?

Measuring your waist will help you find out where you are in relation to where you should be. In general, a woman would try to maintain a waist of 31.5 inches or less and a man should aim for 37 inches or less. Now, this can vary a little and there are BMI charts and indexes you can research. You also have to make sure you are measuring your waist correctly. In order to do so, place the tape measure around your waist starting where it is the narrowest, between the bottom of your rib cage and your hipbone. Have someone help you if needed. The measuring tape needs to be snug, but don't tighten it up too much, and breathe out before you measure.

For women, a measurement of 35 inches and more is concerning. For a man, 40 inches or more is also concerning. You can also look at the waist-hip ratio to complete your assessment. To calculate this ratio, measure first your hips in the largest area of your body—usually around your buttocks. Then take your waist measurement and divide it by this new number. Keep in mind that women should strive to keep below 0.80 and men below 0.95.

HOW MANY CALORIES DO I NEED TO EAT A DAY TO LOSE MY BELLY FAT?

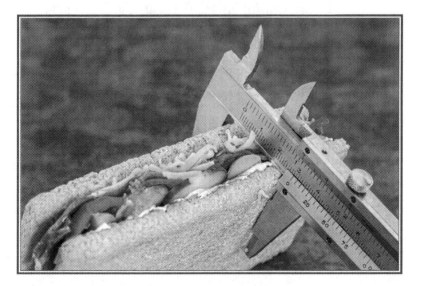

This will vary among individuals depending on multiple factors including activity level. On the average, people should generally keep their caloric intake to somewhere between 1500-2000 calories per day. Remember though, simply speaking your goal should be to burn more calories than you consume, on a macro and micro level. It's also important to mention again that your goal is not to lose weight rapidly but consistently—1 to 2 pounds a week is a good amount. Don't forget that calories are simply a measure of energy. So, if you follow a healthy diet as suggested early on in the book, you will be able to eat until you are satisfied, but the calories you will ingest will be digested appropriately by your body and not stored as fat. Cutting as few as 100 calories per day in your diet can help you lose weight progressively and help you trim that belly down.

AREN'T' MEN SUPPOSED TO HAVE A BELLY ANYWAY?

As hard as it is to believe, some people still believe this, but this is completely wrong. Regardless of whether you are a man or a woman, excess fat in your abdominal area can have very negative consequences on your health. As mentioned before, men may have a predisposition to gain weight in the belly area, and this becomes increasingly true as they get older. This is due to the muscle mass decreasing and when combined with lack of exercise, maintaining a healthy weight can be extremely challenging. So, the fat cells will have to be stored somewhere, and running out of room in the legs and arms, they usually will end up in the belly area.

Let's talk about the notorious beer belly for a moment. It honestly does not matter where the calories contributing to your belly fat come from. But alcohol, including beer, can easily wrack up your daily caloric intake quickly, and decreasing alcohol use is a good idea. If you still want to drink beer, drink it in moderation and switch to light beer. Also, take into consideration that excess alcohol use can lead to more serious health risks such as high blood pressure and liver disease. It also greatly hampers your motivation and makes it nearly impossible to get good and healthy sleep. So it can directly lead to extended periods of inactivity, on top of being high in calories.

IS LIPOSUCTION A VALID SOLUTION TO ELIMINATE BELLY FLAT FOR GOOD?

Liposuction is a medical procedure which slims and shapes certain areas of the body by removing excess fat deposits. You might be dreaming of that 'six pack' some men proudly display or that extra flat belly women like to show off at the beach. You might be discouraged because losing weight in a specific area can sometimes be difficult and most importantly requires serious and dedicated efforts on your part. So, here you are, thinking about going under the knife to look and feel better. But is this a good idea and is it worth spending the significant amount of money?

Liposuction is without a doubt a popular surgery. However, there are several things to consider before you choose to undergo the surgery. After the surgery, if you continue to live a lifestyle where you do not eat sensibly, exercise regularly, or take care of yourself, you will most likely gain back the weight and your belly will be rounded again. The liposuction will certainly help removing some excess fat initially, but the fat around your internal organs, deeper inside will stay.

Chapter 6
MYTHS ABOUT FLAT BELLY

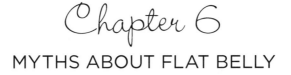

MYTH 1: ALL YOU NEED TO DO TO GET A FLAT BELLY IS ABDOMINAL EXERCISES

False. Abs exercises will help your abdominal muscles to become stronger. However, the fat that you have accumulated over the years is located all the way around the mid-section. So this is not enough. You also need to follow a healthy diet and incorporate in aerobic or cardiovascular exercise into your life.

MYTH 2: EXERCISING YOUR ABS SHOULD HURT

Absolutely false. It should not be painful to exercise, period. Yes, you might experience a little discomfort at first, because your muscles need to get used to the new activities. However, you should always be able to walk normally and go on with your daily activities after exercising. There is always a danger of over- doing it in the gym though. So you need to be sure to keep your routines sensible and increase them over time. Certainly you can be tired, but if you are experiencing strong pain, you may not be exercising correctly.

There is so much free information online regarding different exercise routines and styles, as well as fitness instructors at every gym, that you should not be without ample resources available to assist you.

MYTH 3: FASTING OR SKIPPING MEALS IS THE BEST WAY TO GET A FLAT STOMACH

Also false. Actually neither will help you lose weight in the long run. Not only can this be dangerous to your health, but if you don't eat meals regularly, you will disrupt your body's metabolism causing it to guard your stores of fat. Starving yourself will not get you anywhere but frustrated and sick. Eat more healthy meals in smaller portions. Don't make the mistake of ever thinking that not eating is the key to losing weight anywhere on your body including your tummy.

MYTH 4: DIET PILLS ARE THE WAY TO GO

False. Take a pill every day and don't worry about eating too much, exercising, or gaining weight! Easy right? Unfortunately, it doesn't work that way, and anything that seems that easy has to come with very negative consequences. As we said before, trimming down your belly fat can happen if you combine cardio and healthy diet. You cannot obtain anything that instantaneous and that does not require any effort. Also be very careful. A lot of those supplements are not controlled or regulated by the FDA, so individual side effects may not be known. So if you do opt for this route you should definitely consult with your primary care physician. A recent FDA study found that nearly 70 percent of diet pills are spiked with dangerous substances, and taking diet pills has long been known to potentially cause high blood pressure or even strokes in some individuals. There is nothing easy about 'safely' losing that fat in your abdominal area, which just makes it so much more rewarding when you achieve it.

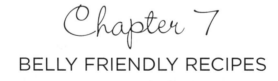

BELLY FRIENDLY RECIPES

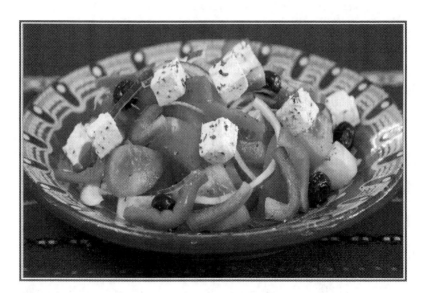

We have already talked about eating habits you should adopt
and foods you should favor. Now, if you are out of options or
getting bored, or just feel like trying some different recipes,
this chapter will make your life much easier. Don't forget to

be creative and modify the recipes slightly to make them to your taste.

SANDWICH IDEAS

Sandwiches are certainly quick and easy meals. And because we suggested that cut down your daily carb intake, it does not mean that you need to eliminate all types of breads or grains completely from your diet. Pita breads, tortillas and lettuce wraps are excellent choices, as they contain less calories. Just make sure you select the whole grains options.

To avoid using mayonnaise which is very high in fat, try different substitutes, such as balsamic vinegar, hummus, or even Greek yogurt with garlic.

Any of the ideas below can keep your menu interesting and help you avoid getting bored eating the same type of sandwiches day in day out:

- *Use chicken breast with a few avocado slices*
- *Mix in tuna with Greek yoghurt, fresh dill, a few slices of cucumbers, onions, pepper*

- *Cook some fresh tilapia with tomatoes, garlic and cilantro*

- *Utilize turkey bacon to make the perfect BLT*

- *Make sure you vary the greens you use on the sandwiches (iceberg, arugula, kale, spinach)*

- *Use olive tapenade on your sandwich for a change*

- *Spread some homemade pesto on your toasted turkey breast*

BREAKFAST'S IDEAS

Breakfast is an extremely important meal. However, many of us are in a hurry in the morning before work, school or dropping off the kids. This is no excuse to skip this meal, or any other meal as a matter of fact.

Try one of the following simple ideas:

- *Cottage cheese with pineapple chucks*

- *Blueberries with Greek yogurt sprinkled with granola*

- *Oatmeal with cinnamon*

- *Smoothies (almond milk, strawberries, bananas- or your favorite fruits and flax seeds)*

- *Boiled egg and a few slices of avocados on a whole grain toast (no butter)*

SMART NACHOS

Remember you can add whatever ingredients you like on the typical dishes you are used to preparing and eating. Use some baked tortilla chips, and any low fat shredded cheese (sharp cheddar, Monterey jack, ricotta, or other). Sauté your favorite vegetables slightly in olive oil and spices for nachos: peppers, onions, mushrooms, scallions. Add some fresh condiments of your choice: tomatoes, cilantro, fat free sour cream, and fresh salsa.

If you want to add meat to your nachos, consider choosing some lean cuts: ground turkey or chicken breast. You can also substitute the meat by simply added some seasoned black beans.

GREEN DELISH BLEND

Don't deprive yourself from raw vegetables just because you are not a big fan of their taste. Prepare a healthy dip to help you gobble up fresh produce. This recipe can be modified to please the whole family by adding your favorite herbs or veggies.

- 1/2 cup fresh basil leaves
- 1/4 cup fresh parsley and ¼ cup of chopped scallions
- 1/4 cup plain fat-free Greek yogurt or fat free sour cream
- 2 tablespoons olive oil or coconut oil
- 1 tbsp. rice vinegar
- 1 teaspoon anchovy paste (or a few tbsp. of capers)
- salt and pepper
- cayenne pepper
- 2 cups of spinach or watercress

Simply pour all the ingredients in your blender, until the consistency is smooth. Refrigerate overnight and serve with your favorite raw vegetables.

LEMON & PEPPER CHICKEN

Remember how we talked about the benefits of consuming cayenne pepper? This recipe is an example of how to use this spice in a low calorie but delicious dish.

- 4 skinless chicken tenders
- Pepper cayenne
- Fresh parsley

- Fresh squeezed lemon juice (2)

- 4 tbsp. olive oil or coconut oil

- 2 tbsp. flour

- 2 tbsp. capers

After flouring the tenders, drop them in a preheated skillet with coconut oil or the oil of your choice. Cook 3 or 4 minutes on each side. Then add lemon juice, parsley and capers. Bring the sauce to boil and let it simmer after for a few additional minutes. Add the pepper cayenne.

Serve the chicken on brown rice and with a side of dark green leafy vegetables.

YUMMY COCONUT SALMON

Salmon and tuna are some of the best fish you can eat. Make sure you bake or grill them instead of frying them to keep their healthy properties untouched. This recipe will serve 4 people.

- 4 fresh salmon fillets

- coconut oil and sesame oil

- 3 garlic cloves

- 2 chopped green onions
- ¼ cup Tamari sauce
- 1 pound of chopped mushrooms
- A few bell peppers, red, orange or yellow- your preference
- 1 bag fresh spinach
- salt and pepper

Preheat oven at 450 °F.

It is better to have two different baking pans to make this recipe. One will be for the salmon and the other one will be for the vegetables.

First of all, prepare the marinade by combining in the blender the tamari, oils, onions and garlic. Then generously brush the sauce on the salmon.

Combine the spinach, peppers and mushrooms in a bowl and pour the remaining sauce on it.

Place the vegetables and the salmon in their respective pans and bake everything for about 15 minutes. Once cooked, season with salt and pepper.

CHEESE & LEMON DELIGHT

This book would not be complete without at least one dessert suggestion. Because you are watching your eating habits and trying to lose weight, it does not mean that you need to deprive yourself completely of sweets. You can learn to cook healthier desserts. It is possible. First of all, make your deserts homemade, all the time. When you buy cakes, cookies or any other baking goods in the store, you will notice that the ingredients used are not in your recommended list of foods. The famous Dr. Oz suggested a healthy 5-layer raspberry cake, I will suggest something simpler and possibly as delicious. Try it!

- 1 cup fat free Greek yogurt
- 1/2 cup low-fat cream cheese (softened)
- 1 cup fresh blueberries or raspberries (your taste)
- The juice and zest of one lemon
- 2 tbsp. of coconut sugar
- 1/4 cup of chopped pecans

Mix vigorously the cream cheese, yogurt, lemon juice, zest and sugar until it becomes creamy and smooth.

Using some clear cups or deep bowls, layer the yoghurt and cheese mix, alternating with nuts and berries. Sprinkle with additional nuts or berries if you like.

CONCLUSION

Now that you have read some tips on how to lose that belly fat, you are ready to start your journey towards a healthier you. Remember that you should always try to obtain results naturally. This means that you should avoid taking over the counter diet pills. These can potentially be very dangerous, and can disrupt your metabolism, by giving you short term results without requiring you to truly change your lifestyle.

Instead, adopt new eating habits, as described in the book. Along the way, you will develop your own favorite recipes, and continue to educate yourself on how to eat healthy. Remember! Eating well, doesn't mean depriving yourself of flavorful foods. Choose fresh ingredients, avoid processed foods, and do not skip meals. Make sure you are always choosing healthy choices, no matter where you eat: restaurant, work, and home. Prioritize certain foods as you learn what will maintain the right number of hormones in your body. Avoid stress as much as possible, because with stress, it will only increase the production of cortisol (the hormone that carries extra fat to your belly when overstimulated), and get enough sleep!

On top of modifying your eating habits, you have learnt that it is also essential that you incorporate exercising into your life. By being active on a regular basis, you will ensure that you ideally burn the calories you take in, and transform them into muscle. Many exercises will help you slim your waist and strengthen your abdominal muscles, such as sit ups, crunches and plank exercises on top of regular cardiovascular activity. Make sure you pick activities that you enjoy, so you can practise them consistently without feeling so much like you are doing a chore. Finally, prioritize sleep in your life. Getting enough sleep is crucial to keep your weight and belly down. Your body needs to be rested in order to function well.

By aiming for a flatter belly and losing weight, you will decrease your chances of developing many medical conditions and even life-threatening diseases. So yes, lose weight by eating well and exercising more to obtain a flat abdominal area. But also do it to live a longer, happier, and healthier life.

CHECK OUT OTHER BOOKS

- Belly Fat Diet for Dummies Kindle Edition

by Erin Palinski-Wade (Author)

- Belly Fat Blast: 7 Underground Secrets I Used to Get Rid of Stubborn Belly Fat Forever Kindle Edition

by Lacey Thompson (Author)

- From Belly Fat to Belly Flat: How Your Hormones Are Adding Inches to Your Waist and Subtracting Years from Your Life -- the Medically Proven Way to Reset Your Metabolism and Reshape Your Body Paperback – November 27, 2007

by C.W. Randolph M.D. (Author), Genie James (Author)

- The Abdominal Exercises Bible: Ab Exercises for Core Strength And A Flat Belly (flat belly, abs, abdominal, exercise workout Book 1) Kindle Edition

by Anholt (Author)

- Flat Belly Recipes: Delicious Weight Loss Recipes for a Flat Belly Kindle Edition

by Avery Scott (Author)

- The Flat Belly Diet: Simple and Delicious Recipes to Help You Lose Weight, Burn Belly Fat and Stay Healthy (Flat Belly Cookbook) Kindle Edition

by Jessica Meyer (Author)

- 6 proven ways to lose belly fast

Naturalnews.com

Printed in the United States
by Baker & Taylor Publisher Services